Caroline Creager's
AIROBIC
BALL™
STRENGTHENING
WORKOUT

CAROLINE CORNING CREAGER, P.T.

EXECUTIVE PHYSICAL THERAPY INC.
BERTHOUD, COLORADO

Library of Congress Card Catalog Number: 94-90684
Creager, Caroline Corning
    The Airobic Ball™ Strengthening Workout
    Creager, Caroline Corning - 1st edition

Executive Physical Therapy, Inc.
P.O. Box 1319
Berthoud, CO 80513 USA
(970) 532-2533 or 1-800-530-6878
email: Caroline_Creager@unforgettable.com
www.CarolineCreager.com

Printed in the United States of America
First Printing: November 1994
Second Printing: January 1999

The author has made every effort to assure that the information in this book is accurate and current at the time of printing. The publisher and author take no responsibility for the use of the material in this book and can not be held responsible for any typographical or other errors found. Please consult your physician before initiating this exercise program. The information in this book is not intended to replace medical advice.

ISBN: 0-9641153-1-X
Library of Congress Card Catalog Number: 94-90684

Cover design by Kathy Tracy Designs, Inc.,
    Denver, Colorado.

Book design by Alan Bernhard, Argent Associated, Inc.,
    Boulder, Colorado.

Photos by Marc Nader.

Edited by Caryl Riedel and Raymond Corning.

Cover Photo Hair and Make-up by Cathy Arentz, Blue Hair, Boulder, Colorado.

Distributed by:
Orthopedic Physical Therapy Products
(800)367-7393 or (612)553-0452

About the Author

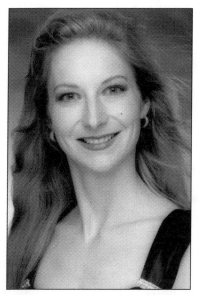

© Marc Nader, 1994

Caroline Corning Creager was born in Richmond, Virginia, and raised in Wasilla, Alaska. She received a Bachelor of Science in Physical Therapy from the University of Montana in 1989. She is the owner of Executive Physical Therapy, in Boulder, Colorado, and is also the author of *The Airobic Ball™ Stretching Workout*, and *Therapeutic Exercises Using the Swiss (Airobic) Ball*. She lectures and teaches seminars throughout the United States promoting the Airobic Ball Stretching and Strengthening Techniques and her modus operandi, "aspire to have a healthy body, not a perfect body."

Dedication

To my husband, Robert, for his nonstop support throughout my numerous projects.

To my brother, Brett Corning, and his family, for making our family feel complete.

To my students at PIMA Medical Institute: Carrie, Heidi, Joe, Linda, Michelle, Monique, Tammy, Thomas, and Tracy. May they be inspired to continue their education and brainstorm new ways to advance their prospective professions.

Acknowledgments

To Barbara and Shari at OPTP, for working so hard to distribute my books.

To Smash, Inc. Aerobic Design Wear by Jill, Greenwood Village, Colorado, for designing my aerobic wear.

To Alan Bernhard, of Argent Associates, Boulder, Colorado, for continuing to help me make the best book possible.

IN MEMORY OF:

Mr. Glen Timmons, and Mr. Ross Carswell,
and all others who lost their lives to cancer.

Table of Contents

THE AIROBIC BALL™ WORKOUT

ARE YOU ONE OF THE MANY AMERICANS who says, "I don't have time to exercise?" When it comes to working out, the majority of Americans would rather watch television, work late, or dream about winning the lottery.

As a physical therapist, I have found that motivating an individual to begin an exercise program that is not enjoyable is very difficult, if not impossible. On the other hand, motivating an individual to begin working out with fun-filled exercises is easily accomplished.

So GET PSYCHED! I have designed an Airobic Ball™ Workout that is fun, challenging, and motivating. You will learn to leave your procrastinating thoughts behind and have a ball while working out on the Airobic Ball™.

Why is the Airobic Ball™ Workout so alluring? Well, as children we grew up playing ball—bouncing, throwing, and kicking balls. No wonder, as adults, the thought of bouncing on an Airobic Ball™ is so fascinating. The Airobic Ball™ Workout provides over 30 strengthening and toning exercises to reshape your abdomen, arms, back, neck, buttocks, and, last but not least, your legs. Unlike conventional fitness programs, the Airobic Ball™ Workout allows you to gain strength, lose weight, AND improve posture, balance, and coordination— all at the same time.

1

THE BEST KEPT SECRET

ORIGINALLY, LARGE, INFLATABLE BALLS were used in the 1960s by Swiss physical therapists to help children with cerebral palsy improve their balance, reflexes, and strength. Now physical therapists and other health care professionals from around the world are teaching the general public and their clients how to break away from traditional fitness regimens and explore new strengthening, stretching, and aerobic exercises using the Airobic Ball™.

Joan Rivers reported on her late night show that the exercise ball is the workout of the "rich and famous." Liz Brody, Associate Editor for *Shape Magazine*, states that "We at *Shape* are willing to bet that axling balls (Airobic Balls™) become one of the next major fitness crazes—at home and in health clubs." (The Airobic Ball™ has also been coined the: **Gymnic Ball**, Axling Ball, and Swiss Ball.)

Mackie Shilstone, M.A., M.B.A., the performance and nutrition consultant to the San Francisco Giants baseball team, St. Louis Blues hockey team, and to over 500 individual professional athletes, has been using Airobic Balls™ to improve the athletes' dynamic balance and proprioception (dynamic postural control) as well as development of specific movement patterns that mimic game situations. Riddick Bowe, a heavyweight professional boxer, is one of the elite athletes Mackie has trained on the Airobic Ball™.

WHY IS THE AIROBIC BALL™ WORKOUT SO UNIQUE?

THE AIROBIC BALL™ IS LIGHTWEIGHT and very portable. You can do this workout just about anywhere: at home, on the job, in the gym, or even in a hotel room while on a business trip or vacation.

The round, mobile surface of the Airobic Ball™ requires dormant muscles to be activated. Just sitting on the ball contracts muscles throughout your body to prevent you from rolling off the ball. When exercising with the Airobic Ball™ your muscles contract in an eccentric manner, which promotes strength gains in a minimal amount of time.

Most exercise programs available today are not designed for both the out-of-shape/overweight and the in-shape/athletic groups. The Airobic Ball™, however, is appropriate for all fitness levels.

BENEFITS OF THE
AIROBIC BALL™ WORKOUT

THE AIROBIC BALL™ BENEFITS are almost too numerous to list. All of the exercises in this book help to improve strength, posture, coordination, flexibility, balance, and endurance. A few additional benefits are:

- Provides a total body workout: abdomen, back, buttocks, chest, inner and outer thighs, legs, shoulders, and neck.
- Burns fat.
- Helps develop body awareness.
- Improves posture and helps align the spine.
- Reduces stress and anxiety.
- Makes bones stronger by improving bone mineral content.
- Improves cardiovascular endurance and helps nourish the discs in the back through the bouncing movements sustained while exercising on the Airobic Ball™.
- Provides a low-impact workout that does not cause undue stress on individual body parts.
- Requires inexpensive equipment and facilities.
- Provides entertainment for the entire family: adults enjoy working out on the Airobic Ball™, newborns love to be bounced to sleep on the Airobic Ball™, and children love to play with Airobic Balls™.

Determining
the Appropriate
Airobic Ball™ Size

Ideally, if you are sitting on the ball with feet flat, the hips and knees should form a 90-degree angle with each other. This sitting position is called the 90-degree rule for sitting.

The following serves as a guideline for determining the appropriate ball size for individuals who exercise in a sitting position:

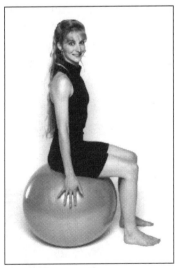

20–25 cm. ball	for non-sitting exercises requiring a small ball
30 cm. ball	children 1 – 2 years old
45 cm. ball	< 5 ft. 0 in. tall
55 cm. ball	5 ft. 0 in. to 5 ft. 7 in. tall
65 cm. ball	5 ft. 8 in. to 6 ft. 3 in. tall
75 cm. ball	> 6 ft. 3 in. tall

Ball size is not only determined by your height, but also by your weight and intended exercise position (sitting, lying on your back, standing, etc.). If you are 5 ft. 6 in. tall and weigh 250 pounds, I recommend the use of a 65 cm. ball. However, if you are 5 ft. 8 in. or shorter and have very short legs, you may want to try using a 55 cm. ball.

What can you do if the Airobic Ball™ you purchase is bigger in diameter than the above guidelines? The answer is, don't inflate your ball as much. For example, if you purchase a 65 cm. ball and are only 5 ft. 2 in. tall, fit the ball using the 90-degree rule in sitting. If your ball is underinflated the ball will not be as firm but you will continue to reap the benefits of the Airobic Ball™.

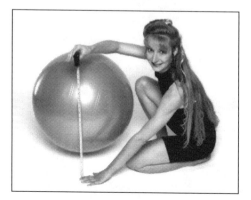

PROPER INFLATION
TECHNIQUES

Allow the ball to reach room temperature before inflating. The balls inflate to a variety of maximum diameters (i.e., 45 cm., 55 cm., etc.) and the maximum diameter is usually printed on the ball. The differing ball diameters allow inflation of balls to approximately the same firmness. It is imperative that the recommended maximum diameter for a given ball size not be exceeded, however, under-inflating the ball is perfectly acceptable.

Many methods are available for inflating the Airobic Ball™:

1. Air compressor
2. Hand pump
3. Foot pump
4. Raft pump
5. Air mattress pump
6. Tire pump with a trigger nozzle adapter

Using an air compressor is the easiest way to inflate a ball. The air compressor forces compressed air into the ball, quickly inflating even the largest ball. Be careful not to over-inflate the ball.

Hand, foot, raft, and mattress pumps are inexpensive and can be purchased for home use. Many of these pumps can be found at a local hardware store, or from the company that sells the Airobic Ball™. Tire pumps at local gas stations can be used in conjunction with a trigger nozzle adapter to inflate balls. Bicycle pumps are inefficient and not powerful enough to properly inflate the balls. Blowing up the balls by mouth, like the use of a bicycle pump, is also ineffective.

Every three to four months Airobic Balls™ may require additional air. If the balls are used extensively, you may need to add air even more frequently.

HOW TO MEASURE THE DIAMETER OF THE AIROBIC BALL™

T O MEASURE THE DIAMETER OF THE BALL, use a tape measure to measure a distance of 55 centimeters (or the appropriate maximum diameter for each ball) up on a wall, beginning at floor level. Put a pencil mark on the wall at the specified height. Then, inflate the ball up to the pencil mark, using a leveled yardstick to span the distance from the mark on the wall to the center of the ball.

AIROBIC BALL™ STRENGTH TRAINING GUIDELINES

THIS WORKOUT IS DESIGNED to strengthen every major muscle group. Strengthening only a few muscle groups at a time may lead to muscle imbalances. A muscle imbalance occurs when one muscle such as the quadricep muscle (front thigh muscle) is a lot stronger than the hamstring muscle (back thigh muscle). Muscle imbalances tend to increase the risk of injury.

Strength training with the Airobic Ball™ will help develop lean, mean muscle mass and burn additional calories. In order for the body to maintain muscle, it requires more oxygen and burns more calories than fat. So the more muscle you have, the more quickly you burn calories, and the faster your metabolism works at play and at rest.

I recommend that you do the Airobic Ball™ Strengthening Workout three to four times per week with at least one day off between workouts. Muscle strength actually improves more rapidly when rest periods of approximately 48 hours (or until muscle soreness is gone) between workouts is used.

Many professional body builders work out every day, but they do not work the same muscle groups. For example, body builders may strengthen their upper body and abdominal muscles on Monday, Wednesday, and Friday, and strengthen their lower body and back on Tuesday, Thursday, and

Saturday. This schedule allows each muscle group 48 hours of rest.

You then have several workout schedule options:

1. Do all 32 Airobic Ball™ exercises at each workout session and work out every other day.

2. Strengthen your upper body and abdomen one day and your lower body and back the next day. A suggested workout schedule is listed below:

MONDAY & FRIDAY

Upper Body and Abdominal Workout

1. Pelvic Tilt Forward and Backward*
2. Waist Trimmer*
3. Pelvic Circles*
4. Arm Circles
5. Jumping Jacks
6. Upper Abdominal Crunch with Arm Push
7. Lower Abdominal Crunch
8. Upper Abdominal Crunch
9. Oblique Abdominal Curl
10. Head and Neck Curl
11. Upper Body Strengthener
12. Prone Walkout
13. Push-Up
14. The Skier
15. Scissor Twist
16. Shoulder Strengthener
17. Wall Push-Up

TUESDAY & SATURDAY

Lower Body and Back Workout

1. Pelvic Tilt Forward and Backward*

* These are good warm-up exercises for both the upper and lower body workout.

2. Waist Trimmer*
3. Pelvic Circles*
4. The Sitting Lunge
5. Glut Lifts – Beginner or Advanced
6. Leg Push/Pull
7. Inner and Outer Thigh Trimmer
8. Inner Thigh Trimmer
9. The Bridge
10. The Bridge: Knee Lift
11. The Bridge: Leg Lift
12. The Back Strengthener
13. Standing Squat
14. Toe Raises
15. Front Squats
16. Standing Ball Toss and Squat
17. Standing Lunge

I will now explain what exercise set and repetition mean. A set is a specific number of repetitions completed without a rest break. A repetition or rep is actively completing one exercise technique. For example, Exercise #17, Standing Lunge, suggests you do the exercise for two sets, with 6 – 10 reps. This means you should do the exercise 6 – 10 times, rest, then repeat the same exercise 6 – 10 times. (I recommend that you take a 20-second rest break between each exercise set.)

I have given you the option of 6 – 10 reps, because many individuals will only be able to do 6 reps, while others will be able to do up to 10 reps. Please refer to the section entitled LISTEN TO YOUR BODY on page 14.

---

* These are good warm-up exercises for both the upper and lower body workout.

THE FLOW SHEET

I HAVE PROVIDED A FLOW SHEET at the end of the book so that you may record your progress on the number of sets and repetitions of each exercise completed, along with your daily exercise heart rate. An example is provided on page 62 to show you how to fill out the flow sheet correctly. By recording your sets, repetitions, and resting heart rate you can follow your weekly progress at a glance.

LISTEN TO YOUR BODY

MANY TIMES WHEN BEGINNING an exercise program, we forget to listen to our bodies. For example, Jennifer is 40 pounds over weight and has not worked out consistently for the last 10 years. She begins doing push-ups (see page 49) for the first time. The book says to repeat the exercise two times, with 8–12 reps each. Jennifer thinks that since the book says to do this exercise 16–24 times, *she* should do the exercise 24 times as well. WRONG! This book only gives guidelines — that means — listen to your body! If your body is tiring after the first repetition, then STOP after the fifth repetition. Rest for at least thirty seconds, and REPEAT a second set of five reps. With time, Jennifer will be able to attain the stated guideline and more. Design your Airobic Ball™ program to meet the individualized needs of your own body. **Adapt the exercise to your body. Do not adapt your body to the exercise.**

STRETCHING

PROPER STRETCHING TECHNIQUES ARE ESSENTIAL for preventing muscular imbalances caused by exercise, work, or other activities of daily living. Stretching increases muscle length, restores circulation, and promotes relaxation.

To safely and effectively increase muscle length, follow these instructions:

1. Avoid bouncing.

2. Slowly stretch within a level of tolerance, not pain.

3. Do not hold your breath. Try to breathe with the exercise.

4. Repeat a stretch three to five times.

5. If appropriate, repeat a stretch in opposite directions, so both sides are stretched equally.

Please refer to *The Airobic Ball™ Stretching Workout* to learn new stretching techniques.

AEROBIC EXERCISE

IS STRENGTHENING CONSIDERED an aerobic activity? There are three requirements for an exercise to be considered aerobic:

1. The activity must use large muscles in a rhythmic manner
2. The intensity of the workout must be between 50% – 90% of your maximal heart rate. (Please refer to: HOW TO FIND YOUR TARGET HEART RATE on page 17.)
3. The duration of continuous exercise must be between 15 and 60 minutes.

Yes, strengthening can be considered an aerobic activity, if you maintain your target heart rate for 15 minutes or longer. This program allows for periodic rest breaks between repetitions, therefore I recommend you augment this program with a traditional aerobic exercise program. Walking, running, bicycling, in-line skating, swimming, and cross-country skiing are all excellent aerobic activities.

Regular aerobic exercise, three to four times per week, further enhances your potential to burn fat, improve stamina, and strengthen your heart and lungs.

How to Find Your Target Heart Rate

A T REST, YOUR HEART BEATS MORE SLOWLY than when you are working out. A normal resting heart rate for someone in excellent shape ranges from 40 to 60 beats per minute. For someone who is somewhat of a couch potato or exercises moderately, the normal resting heart rate ranges from 60 to 100 beats per minute.

When exercising, the heart beats faster to pump blood to all of the working muscles. Since your heart is a muscle, as your exercising increases, your heart muscle becomes better toned and more efficient and does not have to beat as hard. In essence, the heart beats more slowly with the same intensity of exercise. For this reason, it is important to record your heart rate during or immediately after exercise.

An easy way to monitor your exercise intensity is to find your Target Heart Rate. You can find your Maximum Heart Rate by subtracting your age from 220. Your Target Heart Rate should be 60% to 80% of your Maximum Heart Rate.

The equation should look like this:

$$220 - \text{AGE} = \text{MAXIMUM HEART RATE}$$

So your Target Heart Rate Range would be between: $.60 \times (220 - \text{Age})$ and $.80 \times (220 - \text{Age})$.

Use this example:

If you are 35 years old, you would calculate the following:

Your Maximum Heart Rate is: $220 - 35 = 185$

Your Target Heart Rate Range is: $.60 \times (220 - 35) = 111$ to $.80 \times (220 - 35) = 148$ beats per minute.

If you are trying to lose weight, maintain your heart rate at 60% of your maximum heart rate (or at 111 beats per minute for this example).

HOW TO TAKE YOUR PULSE

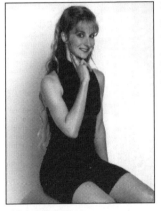

DIAGRAM 1

Y OUR RESTING HEART RATE is most accurate if taken when you first get out of bed in the morning. Your exercise heart rate should be measured during or immediately following exercise. The carotid artery and the radial artery are the two most common sites to find your pulse. Apply light fingertip pressure to the arteries when checking your pulse in order to avoid impediment of the blood supply. The carotid pulse is located by placing the tips of the index and middle fingers (not the thumb as it has its own pulse) just below the jaw bone on the side of your neck (refer to Diagram 1). The radial pulse is found by placing two fingertips on the palm side of your wrist just above the base of the thumb (refer to Diagram 2).

After finding your pulse, start a stopwatch or look at the second hand on a wristwatch. Take your pulse rate for 10 seconds, counting the first beat as zero. To obtain your heart rate in beats per minute (60 seconds), multiply the number of beats you counted by six.

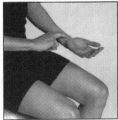

DIAGRAM 2

TRICKS OF THE TRADE

IN ORDER TO STAY IN SHAPE, consistency is the key. Some days you may not feel like exercising, so try to focus on a short-term goal (STG), for example, exercise for 15 minutes instead of 30 minutes. Plan ahead. Think of long-term goals (LTG). What would you like to accomplish in one week, one month, six months or even in a year from now? After you have accomplished your goal, reward yourself with something special — like a monthly massage, an afternoon off from work to go shopping for a new outfit, or allow yourself a week off from cleaning by hiring a cleaning service to do the job. Remember, if you do not adhere to your STG or LTG, you are ineligible for your reward. Here are a few additional tricks of the trade that will help you maintain a lifelong fitness regimen.

1. Schedule your daily workout at the same time of day. If you like to work out in the mornings, try working out every morning at 6:00 am. If you are not an early bird, work out every afternoon at 6:00 pm.

2. Feeling tired and don't want to exercise? Tell yourself you are only going to exercise for 15 minutes, or you're only going to run one mile. Chances are, once you start to exercise, you will complete your full 30-minute program or run an extra mile or two.

3. Hire a professional photographer to take glamorous shots of you. If you make an appointment with a pho-

tographer 3 to 4 months in advance, you will work hard at keeping those muscles in tip-top shape.

4. Manage your exercise program and manage your money. Add one dollar to a jar every time you work out. If you work out five times a week for one month, you will have $40.00 to spend on a new outfit or a new picture for your house.

5. Have custom-fit aerobic wear made for you. Since the workout clothing is made for your body, you look and feel better. Jill Burbary swears you'll look SMASH in her custom-fit aerobic wear. Call (800) OHSMASH for more information.

6. Spoil yourself with a monthly massage. Massages do not have to be expensive. Call a local school of massage and sign up for free or discounted massage. Call the American Massage Therapy Association at (708) 864-0123 for the massage school nearest you.

7. Enhance your beauty with a new hairstyle or with a manicure, pedicure, or facial. Look for a cosmetology school near you where you can receive discounted rates.

8. Are you a chocoholic? Indulge in a mini-chocolate bar.

9. Frustrated with your weight and your eating habits? Consult with a dietitian. Call the American Dietetic Association at (800) 877-1600 for a qualified dietitian near you, your local public health department or hospital.

10. Don't be too hard on yourself if you gain a few pounds back. Just try to remember what may have caused those extra pounds to creep back on. Did you have a stressful month at work or at home? Did you forget to work out? Refocus your energy and reorganize your STGs and LTGs.

HEALTHY EATING HABITS

- Use low-fat dairy products (skim milk, low-fat yogurt, and low-fat cheese).
- Treat yourself to a non-fat yogurt or other non-fat/low-fat dessert and snack.
- Limit egg intake to less than three a week (including those used in cooking). The American Heart Association recommends a daily cholesterol intake of less than 300 milligrams. One egg yolk contains 213 milligrams of cholesterol.
- Substitute two egg whites for one egg yolk when cooking. Egg whites do not contain cholesterol and are a good source of protein.
- Eat more fruits, vegetables, grains, and legumes. These foods tend to be high in vitamins, minerals, and fiber.
- Begin eating whole wheat bread instead of white bread.
- Avoid deep-fat frying. Broil food instead.
- Use cooking oils low in saturated fat. The best choice is a monounsaturated fat such as olive, canola, almond, peanut, or avocado oil.
- Remove skin from poultry (most of the fat in poultry is found in the skin).
- Limit red meat to two times per week.
- Add fish to your diet. Fish is low in calories, cholesterol, and fat.
- Drink lots of water! Water helps curb the appetite and re-plenishes water you lose through perspiration. Drink 8 – 10

eight-ounce glasses of water a day, and an additional glass of water for each 25 pounds of extra weight you are carrying. Water constitutes approximately 57% of your total body weight (Arthur Guyton M.D., 1987). Example: A 115-pound woman's water weight would be approximately 66 pounds.

• Do not try to change poor eating habits overnight. Make a few changes every month and stick with them.

AIROBIC
BALL™
EXERCISES

Pelvic Tilt Forward and Backward

PURPOSE:
To increase flexibility in back and hips.

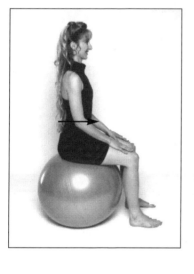

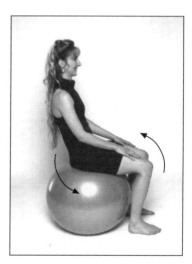

INSTRUCTION:

Sit on ball. Roll ball backward as hips roll forward. Slightly arch back. Return to starting position. Roll ball forward as hips roll backward. Return to starting position.

REPEAT:

2 sets, with 10 – 14 reps

Waist Trimmer

PURPOSE:

To strengthen muscles on sides of waist. To encourage shifting body weight equally from side to side.

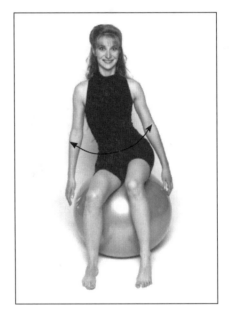

INSTRUCTION:

Sit on ball. Roll ball from side to side by shifting weight from right hip to left hip.

REPEAT:

2 sets, with 10 – 14 reps

Pelvic Circles

PURPOSE:
To increase back and hip flexibility.

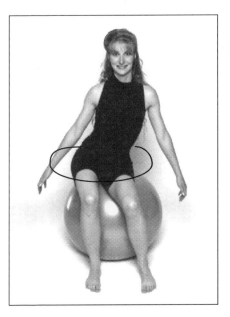

INSTRUCTION:
Sit on ball. Begin drawing a circle, initiating movement from the hips. Rotate the hips clockwise, then rotate the hips counterclockwise.

REPEAT:
2 sets, with 10 – 14 reps in each direction

ALTERNATIVE:
Write the alphabet or make figure eights with your hips.

Arm Circles

PURPOSE:

To strengthen arm and upper back muscles.

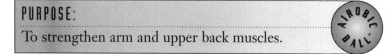

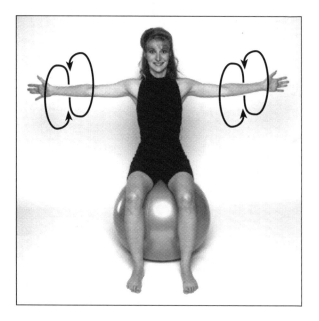

INSTRUCTION:

Sit on ball. Lift arms out away from body with thumbs up.
Rotate arms to make the figure eight.

REPEAT:

2 sets, with 8 – 12 reps

Jumping Jacks

PURPOSE:

To increase range of motion and strengthen
shoulder and leg muscles.

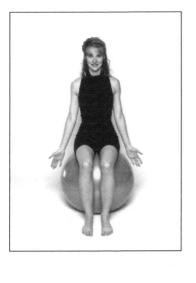

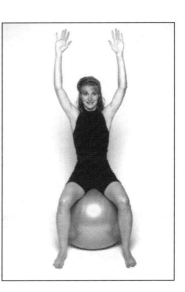

INSTRUCTION:

Sit on ball. Place arms at side of ball. Initiate bounce with
hips. Raise arms overhead and move legs apart. Bounce.
Lower arms to side and move legs together.

REPEAT:

2 sets, with 10 – 14 reps

The Sitting Lunge

PURPOSE:
To strengthen arm and leg muscles.

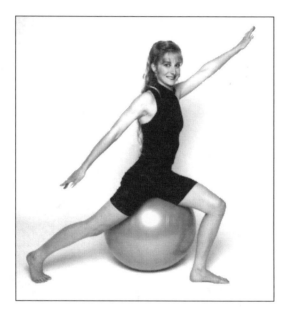

INSTRUCTION:
Sit on ball. Extend arms. Rotate body and extend left leg backward. Keep feet and knees aligned.

REPEAT:
2 sets, with 6 – 10 reps

Glut Lifts — BEGINNER

PURPOSE:
To strengthen leg and buttock muscles.

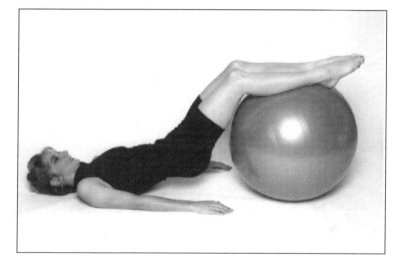

INSTRUCTION:
Lie on back with legs on ball. Lift hips off floor.

REPEAT:
2 sets, with 8 –12 reps

Glut Lifts — ADVANCED

PURPOSE:
To strengthen leg and buttock muscles.

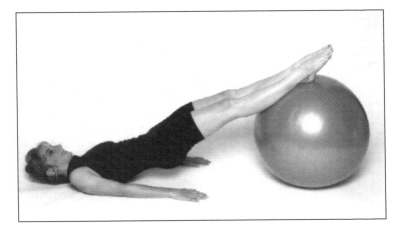

INSTRUCTION:

Lie on back with heels on ball. Lift hips off floor. Keep legs straight.

REPEAT:

2 sets, with 10 – 12 reps

Leg Push / Pull

PURPOSE:
To strengthen thigh and lower leg muscles.

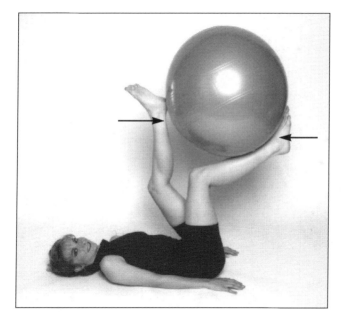

INSTRUCTION:

Lie on back with legs on ball. Place left foot on ball. Push ball with left foot and pull ball toward body with right leg. Hold position for 5 seconds.

REPEAT:

2 sets, with 6 – 10 reps each leg

Upper Abdominal Crunch with Arm Push

PURPOSE:
To strengthen abdominal, mid-back, and neck muscles.

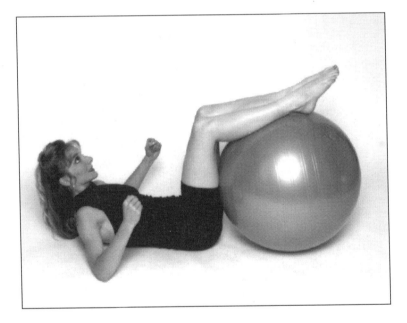

INSTRUCTION:
Lie on back with legs on ball. Bend elbows and move away from body. Raise head and upper body while pushing elbows into floor. Keep eyes focused on ceiling. Return to starting position.

REPEAT:
2 sets, with 8 – 12 reps

Lower Abdominal Crunch

PURPOSE:
To strengthen lower abdominal muscles.

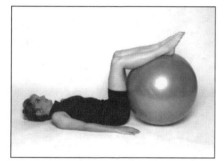

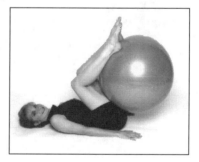

INSTRUCTION:

Lie on back. Bend both knees. Place ball underneath knees. Squeeze ball between feet and legs. Lift ball and knees toward chest.

REPEAT:

2 sets, with 8 – 12 reps

Upper Abdominal Crunch

PURPOSE:
To strengthen upper abdominal muscles.

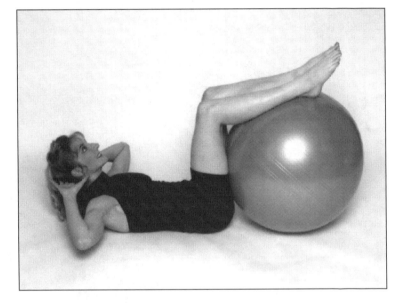

INSTRUCTION:
Lie on back with legs on ball. Place unclasped hands behind head. Raise head and shoulders off floor. Keep eyes focused on ceiling.

REPEAT:
2 sets, with 8 – 12 reps

Oblique Abdominal Curl

PURPOSE:
To strengthen oblique abdominal muscles.

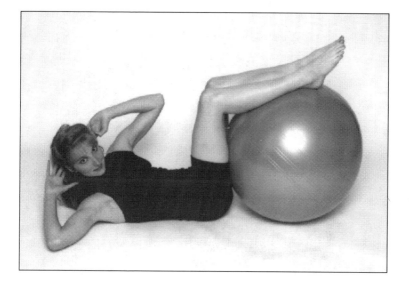

INSTRUCTION:

Lie on back and bend knees. Place unclasped hands behind head. Raise head and shoulders off floor as left elbow rotates toward right knee. Repeat with opposite side.

REPEAT:

2 sets, with 8 – 12 reps

Inner and Outer Thigh Trimmer

PURPOSE:

To strengthen inner thigh, outer thigh, and abdominal muscles.

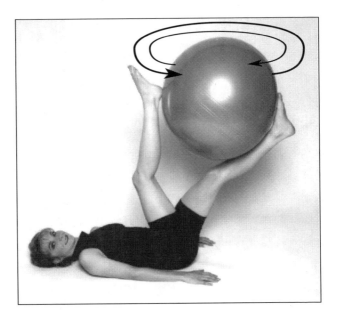

INSTRUCTION:

Lie on back, bend knees, and lift legs toward ceiling. Rotate the ball between feet in both directions.

REPEAT:

2 sets, with 8 – 12 reps

Inner Thigh Trimmer

PURPOSE:
To strengthen inner thigh muscless.

AIROBIC BALL

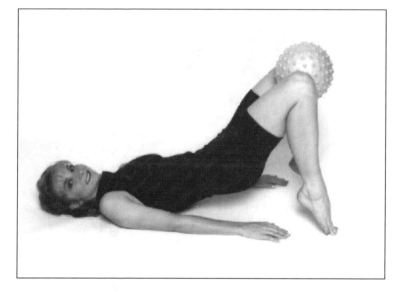

INSTRUCTION:

Lie on back and bend knees. Place small ball between knees.
Flatten back and raise hips and heels off floor while
squeezing ball.

REPEAT:

2 sets, with 12-14 reps

The Bridge

PURPOSE:
To strengthen abdominal, back, and leg muscles.

AIROBIC BALL

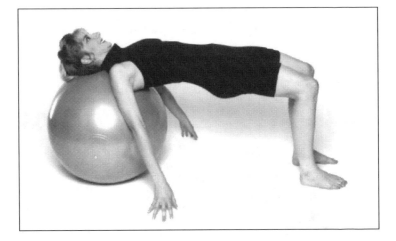

INSTRUCTION:

Sit on ball. Walk legs out away from ball so head and shoulders rest on ball. Body is in a bridge position (see photograph). Rest hands on floor to help with balance. Return to sitting position

REPEAT:

6 – 8 reps

HOLD:

10 seconds each rep

PRECAUTION:

Do not arch back or let buttocks sag.

The Bridge: Knee Lift

PURPOSE:
To strengthen abdominal, back, and leg muscles.

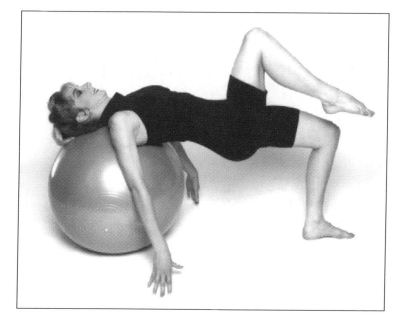

INSTRUCTION:
Lie on ball in bridge position. Rest hands on floor. Raise knee. Return to starting position. Repeat with opposite leg.

REPEAT:
2 sets, with 6 – 8 reps

PRECAUTION:
Do not arch back or let buttocks sag.

The Bridge: Leg Lift

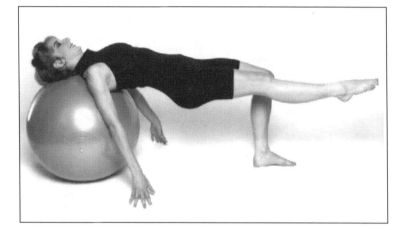

INSTRUCTION:

Lie on ball in bridge position. Rest hands on floor. Extend one leg. Return to starting position. Repeat with opposite leg.

REPEAT:

2 sets, with 6 – 8 reps

PRECAUTION:

Do not arch back or let buttocks sag.

Head and Neck Curl

PURPOSE:
To strengthen neck muscles.

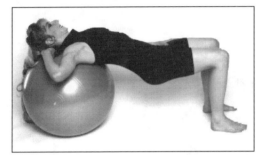

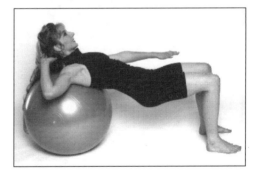

INSTRUCTION:

Begin in bridge position. Let buttocks sag slightly. Place one hand behind head (to support head only). Raise head off ball and reach opposite hand toward knee.

REPEAT:

2 sets, with 5 reps

The Back Strengthener

PURPOSE:

To strengthen back and neck muscles.

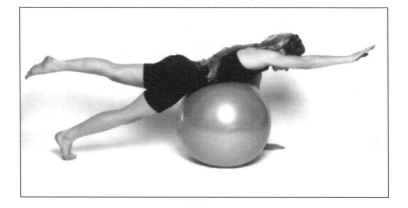

INSTRUCTION:

Kneel. Lie with abdomen on ball. Extend one leg back and opposite arm overhead. Repeat with opposite arm and leg.

REPEAT:

2 sets, with 8 – 12 reps

PRECAUTION:

Do not lift leg or arm so high that back rotates.

Upper Body Strengthener

PURPOSE:
To strengthen arm, upper back, and neck muscles.

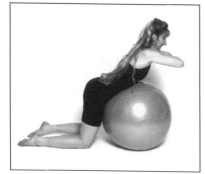

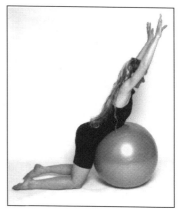

INSTRUCTION:

Kneel. Lean abdomen on ball. Cross hands and place on top of shoulders. Raise arms overhead.

REPEAT:

2 sets, with 6 – 10 reps

Prone Walkout

PURPOSE:
To strengthen arm and shoulder muscles. To improve balance reactions.

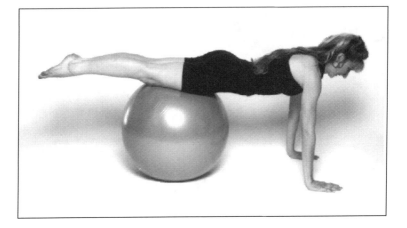

INSTRUCTION:

Kneel. Lie with abdomen on ball. Walk arms out until ball is under thighs.

REPEAT:

2 sets, with 8 – 12 reps

PRECAUTION:

Do not let abdomen sag. Do not round back.

ALTERNATIVE:

Walk arms out until feet are on ball.

Push-Up

PURPOSE:
To strengthen arm muscles. To improve balance reactions.

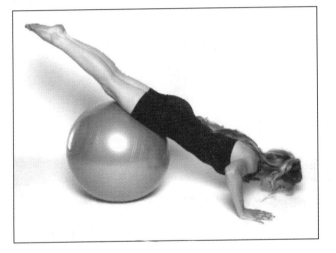

INSTRUCTION:
Kneel. Lie with abdomen on ball. Walk arms out until ball is under thighs. Do a push-up.

REPEAT:
2 sets, with 8 – 12 reps

PRECAUTION:
Do not let abdomen sag.

ALTERNATIVE:
Walk arms out until feet are on ball and do a push-up.

The Skier

PURPOSE:

To strengthen abdominal, arm, back, neck, and hip muscles.

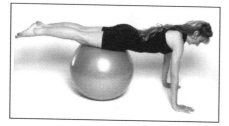

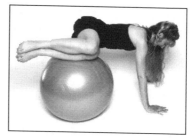

INSTRUCTION:

Kneel. Lie with abdomen on ball. Walk arms out until ball is under thighs. Bend knees and rotate hips so left outer knee is touching ball. Draw knees up to chest on right side. Repeat with opposite side.

REPEAT:

2 reps, with 6 – 10 reps

PRECAUTION:

Eyes should be focused on floor. Maintain head in alignment with shoulders.

The Scissor Twist

PURPOSE:
To strengthen abdominal, arm, back, leg, and neck muscles.

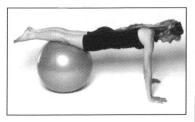

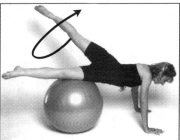

INSTRUCTION:

Kneel. Lie with abdomen on ball. Walk arms out until ball is under thighs. Keep legs straight. Lift one leg up toward ceiling and rotate over opposite leg. Repeat with opposite side.

REPEAT:

2 reps, with 5 – 8 reps

PRECAUTION:

Eyes should be focused on floor. Maintain head in alignment with shoulders.

Standing Squat

PURPOSE:

To strengthen buttock and leg muscles.

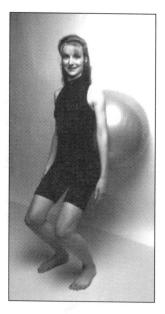

INSTRUCTION:

Stand with feet shoulder-width apart. Place ball between small curve in back and wall. Bend knees.

REPEAT:

2 sets, with 8 – 12 reps

PRECAUTION:

Keep knees aligned over feet when squatting. Do partial squat if unable to do full squat.

Toe Raises

PURPOSE:

To strengthen calf muscles.

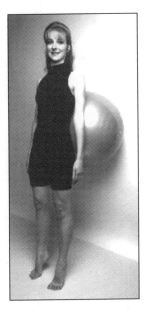

INSTRUCTION:

Stand with feet shoulder-width apart. Place ball between small curve in back and wall. Raise heels off floor.

REPEAT:

2 sets, with 8 – 12 reps

PRECAUTION:

Keep knees bent slightly. Do not lock knees.

Front Squats

PURPOSE:
To strengthen buttock and leg muscles.

AIROBIC BALL

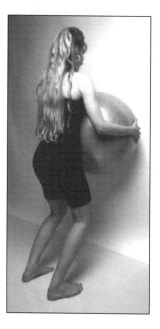

INSTRUCTION:

Stand with feet shoulder-width apart. Place ball between chest and wall and lean into ball. Bend knees.

REPEAT:

2 sets, with 8 – 12 reps

PRECAUTION:

Keep knees aligned over feet when squatting.

Standing Ball Toss & Squat

PURPOSE:
To strengthen buttock and leg muscles. To improve eye-hand coordination.

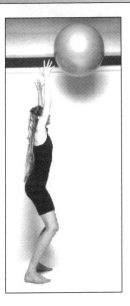

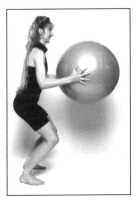

INSTRUCTION:

Stand. Keep eyes and chin level. Toss ball toward ceiling. Squat. Catch ball in squat position.

REPEAT:

2 sets, with 6 – 10 reps

PRECAUTION:

Do not look up at ball when ball is overhead. Eyes should be looking forward at all times.

Standing Lunge

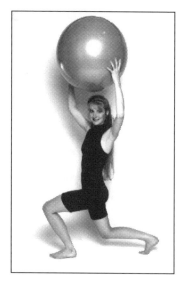

INSTRUCTION:

Stand. Raise ball overhead. Keep eyes and chin level. Lunge forward with left leg. Lower right knee toward floor (do not touch knee to floor). Keep knees aligned over feet. Return to starting position and repeat with opposite leg.

REPEAT:

2 sets, with 6 – 10 reps

REPEAT:

Do not arch back. If unable to lift ball over head without arching back, lower ball until able to do technique properly.

Shoulder Strengthener

PURPOSE:
To strengthen shoulder muscles.

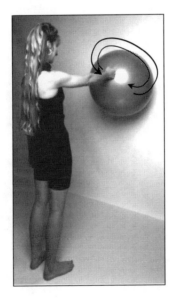

INSTRUCTION:

Stand. Place ball between fisted hand and wall. Straighten arm. Draw a circle initating movement with fist by lightly pressing into ball. Draw circles clockwise for one set and counterclockwise for second set. Repeat with opposite arm.

REPEAT:

2 sets, with 12 – 16 reps

PRECAUTION:

Keep elbow slightly bent throughout exercise.

Wall Push-Up

PURPOSE:
To strengthen arm and shoulder muscles.

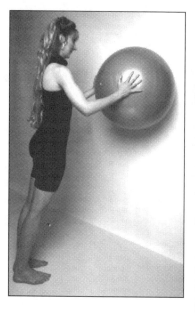
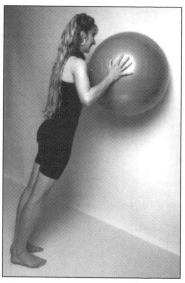

INSTRUCTION:

Stand with feet shoulder-width apart. Place ball between wall and hands. Bend elbows slightly. Do a push-up against ball.

REPEAT:

2 sets, with 8 – 12 reps

REFERENCES

American Heart Association Pamphlet, 1994.

Blair, Steven, et al. *Guidelines for Exercise Testing and Prescription*, Philadelphia: Lea & Febiger, 1986.

Brody, Liz. "Axling: A New Spin on Fitness," *Shape Magazine*, April 1993: pp. 80 – 93.

Creager, Caroline Corning. *The Airobic Ball™ Stretching Workout*, Berthoud, CO: Executive Physical Therapy, 1994.

Creager, Caroline Corning. *Therapeutic Exercises Using the Swiss Ball*, Berthoud, CO: Executive Physical Therapy, 1994.

Duesterhaus, Mary, & Duesterhaus, Scott. *Patient Care Skills*, Norwalk: Appleton & Lange, 1990.

Guyton, Arthur. *Human Physiology and Mechanism of Disease*, Philadelphia: W.B. Saunders, 1987.

Keehan, Jane. "Eccentric Exercise — Delayed Muscle Soreness vs. Training Benefits," *Physical Therapy Forum*, May 13, 1992.

Lockette, Kevin, & Keyes, Ann. *Conditioning with Physical Disabilities*, Champaign: Human Kinetics, 1994.

Pollock, Michael et al. *Exercise in Health and Disease*, Philadelphia: W. B. Saunders Company, 1984.

Rocabado, Mariano, & Antoniotti, Terri. *Exercise and Total Well Being For Vertebral and Craniomandibular Disorders*, Santiago: 1990.

Smith, Craig. "The Warm-Up Procedure: To Stretch or Not to Stretch. A Brief Review," *Journal of Orthopedic Sports Physical Therapy*, 19(1): 12–17, 1994.

SUGGESTED READING

Creager, Caroline Corning. *The Airobic Ball™ Stretching Workout,* Berthoud, CO: Executive Physical Therapy Inc., 1994.

Creager, Caroline Corning. *Therapeutic Exercises Using the Swiss Ball,* Berthoud, CO: Executive Physical Therapy Inc., 1994.

Creager, Caroline Corning. *Therapeutic Exercises Using Foam Rollers,* Berthoud, CO: Executive Physical Therapy Inc., 1996.

Creager, Caroline Corning. *Therapeutic Exercises Using Resistive Bands,* Berthoud, CO: Executive Physical Therapy Inc., 1998.

For more information on ordering these books, please call:

United States/Canada
O.P.T.P.: (800) 367-7393 or (612) 553-0452

Australia/New Zealand
Sport Speed: 61 (02) 6772 7433

United Kingdom
Osteopathic Supplies Limited: 01432 263939

Flow Sheet

Date_____

Date		11/16/94			EXERCISE HEART RATE				EXERCISE HEART RATE			
Exercise	Set	1	2	3		1	2	3		1	2	3
Waist Trimmer	Rep	10	10	–	120							
The Back Strengthener	Rep	12	8	8	–							
	Rep											
	Rep											
	Rep											
	Rep											
	Rep											
	Rep											
	Rep											
	Rep											
	Rep											
	Rep											
	Rep											
	Rep											
	Rep											
	Rep											
	Rep											
	Rep											
	Rep											
	Rep											

Flow Sheet

Name_____

2	3	EXERCISE HEART RATE	1	2	3	EXERCISE HEART RATE	1	2	3	EXERCISE HEART RATE	1	2	3	EXERCISE HEART RATE	1	2	3	EXERCISE HEART RATE	1	2	3	EXERCISE HEART RATE

Ordering Information

To obtain more information about ordering Airobic Balls™, and books, please call the following distributors:

United States/Canada
O.P.T.P.: (800) 367-7393

Australia/New Zealand
Sport Speed: 61 (02) 6772 7433

United Kingdom
Osteopathic Supplies Limited:
01432 263939

OR CHECK US OUT ON OUR WEBSITE:
WWW.CAROLINECREAGER.COM